PANCREATIC CANCER

UNDERSTANDING EVERYTHING IT TAKES

TO HEAL PANCREATIC CANCER

DR. J. WALLER

Contents

INTRODUCTION 3

CHAPTER ONE 5

Hazardous Elements 5

Pancreas Anatomy and Function 9

Pancreatic Cancer Types 14

CHAPTER TWO 19

Hazard Contributors...20

Symptoms and Indications..25

Identification 31

Stage and Outlook...37

CHAPTER THREE 39

Options for Treatment 43

Options for pancreatic cancer treatment could include: 44

Hospice Care 50

Dietary assistance 56

CHAPTER FOUR 63

Survival and Aftercare..63

Strategies for Prevention and Lifestyle 70

Effects on Emotion and Psychology 76

CHAPTER FIVE 79

CONCLUSION 84

THE END 88

INTRODUCTION

One kind of cancer that starts in the cells of the pancreas an organ situated beneath the stomach is called pancreatic cancer. The pancreas produces hormones and enzymes, including insulin, that are essential for digestion and blood sugar management. Aggressive in nature, pancreatic cancer frequently poses difficulties for early identification.

Key features of pancreatic cancer include the following:

Pancreatic cancer types:

Exocrine tumors, which are more prevalent, and endocrine tumors, which include pancreatic neuroendocrine tumors, or PNETs, are the two primary forms of pancreatic cancer. Endocrine cancers grow in the pancreatic cells that produce hormones, whereas exocrine tumors typically originate from the pancreatic ducts.

CHAPTER ONE

Hazardous Elements

Age, family history, smoking, obesity, chronic pancreatitis, and specific genetic disorders are some of the factors that may raise one's risk of pancreatic cancer. Comprehending risk variables is crucial for timely identification and mitigation strategies.

Signs:

In its early stages, pancreatic cancer may not exhibit any symptoms. Abdominal pain, jaundice (yellowing of the skin and eyes), loss of appetite, inexplicable weight loss, and digestive problems are among symptoms that may appear as the condition advances.

Imaging tests including CT, MRI, and endoscopic ultrasonography are frequently used to diagnose pancreatic cancer. It is possible to examine tissue samples for the presence of cancer cells via a biopsy or fine-needle aspiration.

Setting:

Treatment decisions are guided by staging, which establishes the amount of cancer dissemination. Stages of pancreatic cancer are frequently divided into localized (limited to the pancreas) and metastatic (spread to other organs) categories.

Options for Treatment:

Radiation therapy, chemotherapy, targeted therapy, and surgery are possible treatment modalities for pancreatic cancer. The cancer's stage, location, and the patient's general condition all influence the therapy option.

Forecast:

Aggressive in nature, pancreatic cancer frequently has a dismal prognosis. The difficulty in detecting cancer early on adds to the high death rate. The cancer's stage, response to therapy, and general health all affect the prognosis.

Assistive Healthcare:

Supportive care is essential since pancreatic cancer has a significant impact on general health. This covers providing dietary assistance, managing pain, and attending to the psychological and emotional needs of patients and their families.

Current Research:

The goals of ongoing studies and clinical trials are to advance early detection techniques, find novel treatments, and deepen our understanding of pancreatic cancer. Research is now underway to investigate advancements in immunotherapy and personalized medicine.

As a major medical challenge, pancreatic cancer underscores the need for education, research, and a multidisciplinary approach to diagnosis and treatment. For those with pancreatic cancer, early detection and efficient treatment methods are crucial to improve prognoses and general quality of life.

Pancreas Anatomy and Function

With its dual endocrine and exocrine roles, the pancreas is an essential organ that is critical to digestion and blood sugar management. An outline of the pancreas' structure and functions is provided below:

Where:

In the upper abdomen, the pancreas is situated behind the stomach. It is tucked up against the back wall and spans the abdomen horizontally.

Organization:

The pancreas is shaped like an elongated tadpole, which is unusual. The head, body, and tail are its three main components.

The pancreas's body spans the abdomen, its tail goes toward the spleen, and its head is located close to the duodenum, the first segment of the small intestine.

Exocrine Process:

About 95% of the pancreas is devoted to carrying out its exocrine function, which produces digestive enzymes. These digestive enzymes help break down proteins, lipids, and carbs in the small intestine.

The digestive enzymes of the pancreas are amylase (which breaks down carbohydrates), lipase (which breaks down fat), and proteases (which breaks down proteins).

Function of the Endocrine System:

The endocrine function of the pancreas, which includes hormone production, occupies the remaining 5% of its mass. The endocrine cells are arranged into what are referred to as the Langerhans islets.

Insulin and glucagon, the primary hormones generated by the islets of Langerhans, are essential for controlling blood sugar levels.

Insulin

When blood sugar levels rise, beta cells respond by releasing insulin. It lowers blood sugar levels and promotes energy storage by making it easier for cells to absorb glucose.

Glucagon:

Insulin has one effect; glucosegon, released by alpha cells, has the opposite effect. Blood sugar levels rise as a result of stimulating the liver's conversion of stored glycogen into glucose and release of that glucose into the bloodstream.

Regulation of Blood Sugar:

An essential component of preserving blood sugar homeostasis is the pancreas. In order to provide a constant source of energy for the body's cells, insulin and glucagon cooperate to manage blood sugar levels.

Add-on Ducts:

Digestive enzymes are transferred from the pancreatic to the duodenum by means of auxiliary ducts in the pancreas. Prior to entering the duodenum, the auxiliary and main pancreatic ducts converge.

Connection of the Bile Duct:

Shortly before it enters the duodenum, the pancreatic duct connects to the common bile duct. This link enables the liver's generated bile and pancreatic enzymes to be released in unison into the small intestine for effective digestion.

The pancreas has two important roles in the body's metabolism: it is an organ that serves both digestive and endocrine functions. Any impairment to its functioning, whether from illnesses such as pancreatic cancer or insufficiency, can have serious consequences for general health and wellbeing.

Pancreatic Cancer Types

Depending on the kind of cells that the disease starts in, there are several forms of pancreatic cancer. Pancreatic neuroendocrine tumors (PNETs) and exocrine pancreatic cancer are the two primary forms. Below is a summary of each:

Pancreatic exocrine cancer:

Approximately 95% of pancreatic cancer cases are of the exocrine type, which is the most prevalent form. The exocrine cells, which generate digestive enzymes, are where it starts. There are two primary subtypes:

a. Adenocarcinoma of the pancreas (PDAC):

With the majority of instances, this is the most prevalent kind of exocrine pancreatic cancer. It is frequently discovered at an advanced stage and develops from the cells lining the pancreatic ducts.

b. Cancer of the Acinar Cells:

A less frequent subtype of exocrine pancreatic cancer is acinar cell carcinoma. The acinar cells, which generate digestive enzymes, are where it starts. Generally speaking, it has a better prognosis than pancreatic ductal adenocarcinoma.

C. Adenosquamous Carcinoma and Additional Uncommon Forms:

Adenosquamous carcinoma is an uncommon subtype of cancer that combines elements of squamous (squamous cell carcinoma) and glandular (adenocarcinoma) cells. Undifferentiated carcinoma and signet ring cell carcinoma are possible additional uncommon subtypes.

Neuroendocrine tumors of the pancreas (PNETs):

Islet cell tumors, another name for pancreatic neuroendocrine tumors, are a less prevalent kind of pancreatic cancer, making up only 5% of cases. The hormone-producing pancreatic islet cells are the source of these malignancies. PNETs can be further categorized into many categories according to the hormones they generate:

a. Insulinomas:

Insulinomas overproduce insulin, which lowers blood sugar levels (hypoglycemia). Among the symptoms could include weakness, disorientation, and fainting.

b. Gastromatomas:

Excessive production of gastrin by gastrinomas results in elevated generation of stomach acid. Peptic ulcers and other digestive problems may arise from this.

C. Glucagonomas:

Blood sugar levels rise as a result of glucagonomas' overproduction of glucagon. Diabetes, skin rashes, and weight loss are possible symptoms.

d. Somatostatinomas:

Excessive production of somatostatin by somatostatinomas disrupts the balance of many hormones. Diabetes, gallstones, and diarrhea are possible symptoms.

e. VIPomas:

CHAPTER TWO

Vasoactive intestinal peptide (VIP), which is produced by VIPomas, causes severe diarrhea and electrolyte imbalance.

f. Non-Working PNETs:

Some PNETs are regarded to as non-functional since they do not generate appreciable amounts of hormones. These tumors might not produce any particular hormonal signs, and they might be found by accident.

The type of cancer, the patient's general condition at the time of diagnosis, and other factors all affect the prognosis and course of therapy for pancreatic cancer. For pancreatic cancer to be properly managed, early detection and individualized treatment approaches are crucial.

Hazard Contributors

Pancreatic cancer is a multifactorial illness that can be influenced by a number of risk factors. Although the precise etiology of pancreatic cancer is frequently unknown, a number of risk factors have been found to raise the likelihood of the disease occurring. These are a few typical risk factors:

Age:

Most incidences of pancreatic cancer occur beyond the age of 65, and diagnoses tend to occur in older persons. As one gets older, the risk rises.

Smoking:

One of the main risk factors for pancreatic cancer is cigarette smoking. Compared to non-smokers, smokers have a greater risk of developing pancreatic cancer, and this risk increases with prolonged smoking.

Family Background:

Certain genetic disorders or a family history of pancreatic cancer can raise the risk. A increased risk may apply to those who have a first-degree relative (parent, sibling, or child) with pancreatic cancer.

Genetic Mutations Inherited:

The BRCA1, BRCA2, PALB2, and p16/CDKN2A genes are among the inherited genetic variants that can raise the risk of pancreatic cancer. For those with a strong family history, genetic counseling and testing may be advised.

Long-term Pancreatitis:

Over time, pancreatic cancer risk may increase as a result of chronic pancreatitis, or persistent inflammation of the pancreas. Those who have inherited pancreatitis are especially at risk for this.

Diabetes:

Diabetes for an extended period of time, particularly type 2 diabetes, is linked to a higher risk of pancreatic cancer. Diabetes and pancreatic cancer have a complicated association that can involve common risk factors.

Overweight:

Carrying extra weight around the belly is especially associated with obesity and raises the risk of pancreatic cancer. Reducing this risk might be facilitated by maintaining a healthy weight.

Nutritional Elements:

The risk of pancreatic cancer may be influenced by specific dietary factors. An elevated risk has been linked to a diet heavy in processed and red meats and low in fruits and vegetables.

Drinking of Alcohol:

Long-term and heavy alcohol use is thought to increase the risk of pancreatic cancer. Reducing alcohol use could lessen this risk.

Exposures at Work:

Pancreatic cancer risk may rise with exposure to specific occupational dangers, such as chemicals and pesticides. Workers in specific industries might come into contact with these toxins.

Race and Gender:

Men are slightly more likely than women to have pancreatic cancer. In addition, African Americans are more vulnerable than people from other racial or cultural origins.

It is crucial to remember that the presence of one or more risk factors does not ensure the development of pancreatic cancer, and some patients may not have any known risk factors. On the other hand, some people who have risk factors might not ever have pancreatic cancer.

For those who are at risk of pancreatic cancer, routine checkups, early identification, and lifestyle changes can all help lower the risk and improve outcomes. It is advised to speak with healthcare professionals for individualized risk assessments and preventative steps, particularly for people with known risk factors or a family history.

Symptoms and Indications

Early-stage pancreatic cancer symptoms might vary based on the tumor's location and size, often exhibiting no symptoms at all. A variety of symptoms and indicators may appear as the cancer spreads. It's crucial to remember that several non-cancerous illnesses might potentially induce same symptoms. Get medical help right away if any of these symptoms are bothersome or persistent. Following are typical indications and symptoms of pancreatic cancer:

Pain in the abdomen:

Pancreatic cancer frequently manifests as back or upper abdominal pain. The tumor's growth may cause the pain to become more intense.

Greenish-white color:

The yellowing of the skin and eyes is called jaundice. It happens when a tumor blocks the bile ducts, causing bilirubin to accumulate in the blood. Pale-colored feces and black urine are possible symptoms of jaundice.

Unexpected Loss of Weight:

Unexpectedly losing a lot of weight is a common sign of pancreatic cancer. Even if the person isn't making an effort to reduce weight, they might nevertheless lose weight.

Diminished Appetite:

Loss of appetite brought on by pancreatic cancer might result in less food being consumed and weight loss.

Problems with the Digestive System:

Digestional abnormalities could manifest as bloating, indigestion, and trouble digesting fat foods. This may be the result of the pancreas's interruption of the production of digesting enzymes.

Vomiting and nauseous:

Vomiting and nausea are possible, frequently as a result of the tumor interfering with the digestive system's regular operation.

Diabetes that develops for the first time or gets worse already:

Changes in blood sugar levels can result from pancreatic cancer's impact on insulin production. Pancreatic cancer may be linked to either newly developed diabetes or a worsening of pre-existing diabetes.

Weary:

Weakness and widespread exhaustion are typical signs of numerous malignancies, including pancreatic cancer. The effects of the malignancy on general health may cause the body's energy reserves to be depleted.

Greasy, Pale Stools:

Disturbances in the regular processes of digestion can lead to alterations in the color and consistency of the stool, including oily or pale stools.

Abnormalities of Blood Clotting:

Blood coagulation disorders can result in deep vein thrombosis (DVT) or pulmonary embolism, and pancreatic cancer may raise this risk.

Skin Itching:

The accumulation of bile salts in the skin as a result of blocked bile ducts can cause itchy skin even in the absence of an obvious rash.

It's crucial to stress that having these symptoms does not always mean you have pancreatic cancer; they might be brought on by a number of different illnesses. Nonetheless, if symptoms are ongoing or getting worse, a complete medical examination should be performed to identify the underlying reason and start the necessary diagnostic procedures. Pancreatic cancer outcomes can be improved by early detection and care.

Identification

A physical examination, a medical history evaluation, and several diagnostic tests are used to diagnose pancreatic cancer. Pancreatic cancer is commonly identified at an advanced stage because of the deep abdominal location of the pancreas and the lack of early detectable signs. On the other hand, earlier detection and diagnosis of pancreatic cancer are now possible because to developments in imaging and diagnostic methods. The following are crucial steps in the diagnosing process:

Medical Background and Physical Assessment:

In order to evaluate risk factors, symptoms, and any pertinent family history, a complete medical history is acquired. To look for symptoms including jaundice, weight loss, and abdominal pain, a physical examination may be done.

Blood Examinations:

Numerous markers can be evaluated by blood tests, such as bilirubin levels, pancreatic enzyme levels (including lipase and amylase), and liver function tests. Certain indicators may be elevated in cases of pancreatic blockage or dysfunction.

Imaging Research:

Imaging investigations are essential for gaining a visual representation of the pancreas and its surrounding components. Typical imaging investigations consist of:

With the use of a CT (Computerized Tomography) scan, which offers precise cross-sectional images of the pancreas, malignancies can be identified and their size and extent evaluated.

With the use of MRI (Magnetic Resonance Imaging), which provides fine-grained images of the pancreas and surrounding tissues, malignancies and potential involvement of nearby structures can be assessed.

Endoscopic Ultrasound (EUS): This technique visualizes the pancreas, surrounding organs, and lymph nodes by combining endoscopy and ultrasound. EUS enables more accurate imaging and is frequently utilized to guide biopsy procedures.

In order to get X-ray images, endoscopic retrograde cholangiopancreatography (ERCP) involves injecting contrast dye into the bile and pancreatic ducts. Abnormalities and obstructions can be detected by ERCP.

Positron Emission Tomography (PET) scan: This test helps identify whether cancer has spread to other organs by providing information about the body's metabolic activity.

Biopsy of Tissue:

The most common method of confirming a definitive diagnosis of pancreatic cancer is a biopsy, which involves taking a little sample of tissue for analysis. Methods for biopsies could include:

Fine-Needle Aspiration (FNA): Tumor cells are removed for examination using a thin needle.

Core Needle Biopsy: To take a core tissue sample for a more thorough investigation, a bigger needle is employed.

ERCP stands for endoscopic retrograde cholangiopancreatography.

ERCP is a useful procedure that can be used to take tissue samples for biopsy in addition to imaging. The pancreatic and bile ducts are accessed by inserting an endoscope through the mouth into the small intestine.

Genetic Examination:

Genetic testing could be advised if there is a known genetic mutation or a family history of pancreatic cancer. This can assist in determining the risk of pancreatic cancer in inherited forms.

Laparoscopy:

In certain situations, a laparoscopy may be necessary to see the pancreas and its surrounding components up close. Through this minimally invasive surgical approach, the afflicted area can be examined and biopsied.

The combination of various diagnostic modalities aids in the establishment of the diagnosis, ascertains the cancer's stage, and directs treatment choices. The absence of particular symptoms in the early stages of pancreatic cancer makes early diagnosis difficult, which emphasizes the significance of continuing research for better screening techniques and early detection tactics.

Stage and Outlook

Understanding and treating pancreatic cancer require a thorough understanding of its stage and prognosis. The staging process entails assessing the cancer's spread, whereas the prognosis offers insight into the disease's expected trajectory and possible consequences. The TNM approach, which takes into account the tumor's size, lymph node involvement, and the existence of distant metastases, is commonly used to stage pancreatic cancer. This is a synopsis:

Pancreatic Cancer Staging:

Stage 0: In situ carcinoma

The cancer has not spread to deeper tissues; it is limited to the outermost layers of cells lining the pancreatic duct.

Phase I:

IA: The tumor is smaller than 2 cm and is limited to the pancreas.

IB: The tumor is still inside the pancreas, but it is more than two cm in size.

CHAPTER THREE

Phase Two:

IIA: The tumor has not yet migrated to neighboring lymph nodes, but it has infected surrounding tissues or organs.

IIB: The tumor has migrated to neighboring lymph nodes and infected adjacent tissues or organs.

Phase Three:

The cancer has not progressed to distant organs, but it has reached significant blood arteries close to the pancreas.

Phase IV:

The peritoneal cavity, lungs, and liver are among the distant organs where the malignancy has spread.

Pancreatic cancer prognosis:

Pancreatic cancer has an overall survival rate that is relatively poor, and the prognosis is frequently guarded. Numerous factors impact the prognosis:

Cancer Stage:

In general, the prognosis improves with an earlier diagnosis. Regretfully, advanced stages of pancreatic cancer are frequently detected at diagnosis.

Size and Location of Tumors:

The prognosis may be affected by the tumor's location and size inside the pancreas. While tumors in the body or tail may not show symptoms until later on, tumors in the pancreas head may produce problems early.

Participation of Lymph Nodes:

A worse prognosis is linked to the presence of cancer in neighboring lymph nodes, suggesting a greater chance of disease dissemination.

Sterilization Possibility:

With surgical excision, the best likelihood of long-term survival is achieved by removing the tumor. Nevertheless, at the time of diagnosis, a small percentage of pancreatic malignancies can be surgically removed.

Reaction to Medication:

The prognosis may change depending on how the patient reacts to chemotherapy, radiation therapy, and surgery. Those who react favorably to treatment can have better results.

General Fitness and Health:

The prognosis is influenced by the patient's overall health and fitness, including their capacity to tolerate treatment and their dietary status.

Genetic Elements:

The genetic profile may affect the prognosis in cases of certain genetic mutations or hereditary pancreatic cancer.

It's crucial to remember that each person is different and that prognoses might differ greatly. Results are still being impacted by new discoveries in research and treatment options, and current clinical trials are looking into innovative ways to increase the survival and quality of life for people with pancreatic cancer. In order to provide complete care and address the various issues associated with pancreatic cancer, a multidisciplinary strategy comprising oncologists, surgeons, radiologists, and supportive care teams is essential.

Options for Treatment

The complexity of pancreatic cancer therapy is contingent upon a number of elements, such as the cancer's stage, the tumor's location, the patient's general health, and the existence of any underlying medical disorders. To develop a customized treatment plan, a multidisciplinary team comprising radiation oncologists, surgeons, oncologists, and other specialists is frequently engaged.

Options for pancreatic cancer treatment could include:

Surgery:

The gallbladder, part of the bile duct, the head of the pancreas, and a portion of the small intestine are removed during the Whipple Procedure (Pancreaticoduodenectomy). Tumors in the pancreatic head are frequently treated with this surgery.

Distal pancreatectomy: Removes the pancreatic tail and occasionally the entire organ. Tumors in the body or the pancreatic tail are treated with this surgery.

A total pancreatectomy is the removal of the pancreas in its whole. Although less often, this surgery can be required in specific circumstances.

Chemotherapy:

Drugs are used in chemotherapy to either kill or inhibit the growth of cancer cells. It is frequently used to target any remaining cancer cells, reduce tumor size, and enhance surgical outcomes either before or after surgery. For pancreatic cancer, common chemotherapy medications include oxaliplatin, 5-fluorouracil, gemcitabine, and nab-paclitaxel.

Radiation Treatment:

High-energy beams are used in radiation therapy to target and destroy cancer cells. It can be used in conjunction with chemotherapy, before to surgery to reduce tumor size, or following surgery to eradicate any cancer cells that may still be present. The most prevalent kind of radiation for pancreatic cancer is external beam radiation.

Personalized Medicine:

Drugs used in targeted therapy deliberately target certain molecules involved in the development of cancer. Chemotherapy may be combined with targeted medicines, such as erlotinib (Tarceva), for pancreatic cancer.

Immunotherapy:

The goal of immunotherapy is to prime the immune system to identify and combat cancerous cells. Although immunotherapy is not as well-established as it is for certain other malignancies, clinical trials are investigating its potential as a treatment for pancreatic cancer.

Clinical Examinations:

Enrolling in clinical trials advances our understanding of pancreatic cancer while giving patients access to cutting-edge treatments. Research on novel treatments and methods never stops.

Hospice Care:

Palliative treatment is intended for patients with advanced pancreatic cancer with the goals of reducing symptoms, controlling pain, and enhancing quality of life. It can be administered in addition to other cancer therapies.

Assistive Healthcare:

Measures to control symptoms and therapeutic side effects, such as pain management, nutritional support, and emotional support, are included in supportive care. It seeks to enhance the general health of those receiving cancer treatment.

Personalized Health Care:

The ability to identify particular genetic alterations in cancers is made possible by developments in molecular profiling and genetic testing. By using this information to inform treatment choices, targeted medicines that are customized to each patient's unique tumor profile can be used.

It's crucial to remember that each person's unique circumstances determine the best course of action, and treatment regimens may combine these techniques. Furthermore, continuous cooperation between the patient's medical team and the pancreatic cancer management team is frequently necessary to address the patient's changing needs and possible therapy modifications. For those with pancreatic cancer, improved results are attributed to early detection when feasible and availability to all-encompassing care.

Hospice Care

Because pancreatic cancer is frequently identified at an advanced stage and can present with severe symptoms and problems, palliative care is essential to the overall management of the disease. Palliative care addresses the physical, mental, and practical requirements of patients with terrible illnesses, such pancreatic cancer, with the goal of enhancing their quality of life. It should not be confused with end-of-life care. The following are important elements of pancreatic cancer palliative care:

Pain Control:

Severe pain has been linked to pancreatic cancer. Palliative care experts collaborate closely with patients to manage pain using a range of therapies, such as prescription drugs, nerve blocks, and other pain control methods.

Control of Symptoms:

The goal of palliative care is to reduce symptoms like weariness, nausea, vomiting, and appetite loss. Supportive therapies and medications are used to increase general comfort and wellbeing.

Support for Nutrition:

It can be difficult for people with pancreatic cancer to maintain a healthy diet because of things like appetite loss, digestive problems, and weight loss. Nutritional counseling and recommendations for dietary changes or nutritional supplements are given by palliative care teams.

Psychological and Emotional Assistance:

For patients and their families, receiving a pancreatic cancer diagnosis can be extremely taxing. Palliative care helps patients cope with anxiety, despair, and other emotional pressures by offering support groups, psychotherapy, and other forms of emotional and psychological support.

Talking and Making Decisions:

Open and honest communication regarding a patient's prognosis, available treatments, and care objectives is facilitated by palliative care teams. They assist people and families in deciding on their preferred level of care with knowledge.

Help with Real-World Issues:

Beyond just treating medical conditions, palliative care also takes care of practical concerns including financial support, care coordination, and system navigation.

Planning for End-of-Life Care:

Palliative care includes talking about end-of-life care preferences, such as making advance directives or living wills, planning for end-of-life care, and making decisions regarding resuscitation. These discussions aid in guaranteeing that people's desires are honored.

Comprehensive Method:

Palliative care adopts a comprehensive perspective, taking into account a person's physical, emotional, social, and spiritual needs. The overarching goal of this holistic treatment strategy is to improve quality of life.

Assistance for Caretakers:

When it comes to the treatment of patients with pancreatic cancer, caregivers are essential. Palliative care acknowledges the difficulties that caregivers encounter in giving care and emotional support, and it offers tools and assistance for them.

Transitional Hospice Care:

When curative treatments for advanced pancreatic cancer are no longer effective, patients may be placed in hospice care. The goal of hospice care is to comfort and assist patients as they approach death, and hospice care can be smoothly transitioned from palliative care.

When palliative care is used with active cancer treatments early in the course of pancreatic cancer, it is most beneficial. It enhances continuing cancer treatments rather than being restricted to end-of-life care, with the goal of improving the general quality of life for patients and their families. The objective is to offer comprehensive care that takes into account the special requirements and difficulties related to pancreatic cancer.

Dietary assistance

A crucial part of the total care given to patients with pancreatic cancer is nutritional support. Nutritional status may be impacted by pancreatic cancer because of things like appetite loss, weight loss, digestive problems, and trouble consuming enough food. The goals of appropriate nutritional support are to raise vitality, assist the body's ability to deal with the stresses of cancer and its treatment, and promote general health. The following are important facets of pancreatic cancer nutritional support:

Nutritional Guidance:

When it comes to giving patients with pancreatic cancer individualized dietary advice, registered dietitians are essential. Taking into account the patient's symptoms, preferences, and treatment plan, they evaluate nutritional needs, deal with dietary difficulties, and suggest adjustments.

Consumption of Calories and Needs for Protein:

It's critical to maintain a sufficient calorie intake, particularly if weight loss is an issue. To maintain immune system and muscle maintenance, there may be an increase in protein requirements. It could be advised to take nutritional supplements to meet needs for protein and energy.

Little, Regular Meals:

For those with digestive problems or low appetite, eating smaller, more frequent meals throughout the day may be easier to handle. This strategy can support sustaining dietary intake.

Rich in Nutrients Foods:

It is imperative to prioritize nutrient-dense foods in order to guarantee that people get the vitamins and minerals they require. Fruits, vegetables, whole grains, lean meats, and healthy fats are some of these foods.

Drinking plenty of water

Drinking enough of water is crucial, particularly for those who throw up or have diarrhea. Sufficient hydration promotes general well-being and aids with symptom management.

Treatment with pancreatic enzyme replacement (PERT):

Pancreatic enzyme replacement treatment may be recommended for people whose pancreatic cancer has affected their ability to produce digestive enzymes. Through the replacement of enzymes that the pancreas is unable to produce in sufficient amounts, PERT aids in better nutritional absorption and digestion.

Addenda:

Supplements containing vitamins and minerals could be suggested to treat deficits or fulfill certain dietary requirements. Supplements, however, have to be used under a doctor's supervision.

Working Together in a Multidisciplinary Team:

It is crucial for healthcare professionals to work together, including nutritionists, oncologists, and other team members. This guarantees a thorough approach to treating dietary requirements, treatment side effects, and general health.

Handling Symptoms of Digestion:

Nausea, vomiting, diarrhea, or malabsorption are examples of digestive symptoms that people with pancreatic cancer may encounter. Managing these symptoms is part of providing nutritional support in order to enhance the person's capacity to tolerate food.

Keeping an eye on and modifying diet plans:

The way a person responds to treatment, how their symptoms change, and their general state of health should all be taken into consideration while modifying their nutritional programs. Consultations with a dietician on a regular basis are crucial.

Education for Patients and Caregivers:

Effective nutritional assistance requires educating patients and their caregivers about the value of nutrition, possible therapeutic side effects on nutritional status, and food challenge management techniques.

One of the most important components of supportive treatment for patients with pancreatic cancer is maintaining optimum nutrition. Enhancing overall quality of life, bolstering the body's resistance to illness and therapy, and augmenting the efficacy of therapeutic therapies are the objectives. Effective nutritional support involves continual collaboration with healthcare providers, individualized nutritional regimens, and close monitoring.

CHAPTER FOUR

Survival and Aftercare

When discussing pancreatic cancer, "survivorship" refers to the time after active treatment which could include chemotherapy, surgery, or a mix of therapies—has ended. Survivors of pancreatic cancer can benefit from continued care, support, and monitoring for possible recurrence or late effects of treatment, even though the disease presents unique challenges because it is frequently diagnosed at an advanced stage. Key elements of pancreatic cancer survivability and follow-up care are as follows:

Frequent Visits for Follow-Up:

After completing pancreatic cancer treatment, patients usually follow up with their medical team on a regular basis. During these visits, the patient's progress can be tracked, any residual side effects can be evaluated, and ongoing health issues can be addressed.

Imaging and Lab Examinations:

Periodic imaging studies (such as CT or MRI scans) and laboratory testing are frequently part of follow-up care to keep an eye out for any indications of cancer recurrence. These tests aid in the early detection of possible problems.

Handling Treatment's Late Effects:

Treatment side effects must be addressed and managed as part of survivorship care. For those who have survived pancreatic cancer, this may entail managing the long-term side effects of radiation or chemotherapy, keeping an eye on pancreatic function, and treating digestive problems.

Support for Nutrition:

In order to survive, nutritional support is still crucial. Sustaining a nutritious and well-balanced diet can help manage any persistent nutritional challenges and improve general well-being.

Both mental and physical health:

The treatment of survivorship involves attending to their mental and physical health. People may have persistent exhaustion, anxiety, or emotional difficulties as a result of their cancer experience. Counseling, survivorship programs, and supportive care services can all be helpful.

Keeping an eye out for cancer recurrence:

Being alert for any indications of a cancer recurrence is part of survivor care. Frequent examinations and honest communication with medical professionals guarantee that any possible problems are dealt with right away.

Way of Life Suggestions:

Supporting and promoting healthy lifestyle choices is a crucial component of care for survivors. This entails engaging in consistent physical activity, abstaining from tobacco and excessive alcohol use, and embracing additional behaviors that promote good health.

Resources and Support Groups:

For survivors, it's common to establish connections with people who have gone through comparable struggles. Individuals entering the post-treatment phase can benefit from the emotional support and important information offered by support groups, survivorship programs, and resources.

Examining Potential Second Cancers:

Survivors of pancreatic cancer might be more susceptible to getting some other cancers. Therefore, depending on a patient's unique risk factors and medical history, survivorship care may include screening for recurrent cancers.

Genetic Testing and Counseling:

When a survivor's family members are suspected of having a hereditary predisposition to pancreatic cancer, genetic counseling and testing might be advised. This can support the development of effective risk-reduction and surveillance plans.

Planning Ahead for Care:

Continual talks regarding advance care planning, such as living wills, advance directives, and preferences for end-of-life care, are part of survivorship care. These discussions guarantee that people's desires are acknowledged and honored.

Frequent visits to primary care:

Survivors should continue routine primary care visits in addition to their oncology follow-up appointments in order to address general health issues, preventive care, and general well-being.

A thorough, multidisciplinary approach is used in pancreatic cancer survivorship care to address the practical, emotional, and physical aspects of life after treatment. Pancreatic cancer survivors' well-being is influenced by their focus on maintaining a healthy and balanced lifestyle, their adherence to suggested follow-up plans, and their continuous communication with healthcare providers.

Strategies for Prevention and Lifestyle

There are some lifestyle choices and preventative techniques that may help lower the chance of developing pancreatic cancer, even though the precise causes of the disease are not always understood. It's crucial to remember that not all risk factors can be changed, and some people may still get pancreatic cancer even after adopting preventative measures. On the other hand, leading a healthy lifestyle can enhance general wellbeing and possibly reduce the risk. The following are some lifestyle choices and ways to avoid pancreatic cancer:

Give Up Smoking:

One of the main risk factors for pancreatic cancer is cigarette smoking. One of the best ways to lower the risk is to stop smoking. If you smoke, look for tools and assistance to help you stop.

Sustain a Healthy Weight:

There is evidence connecting obesity to a higher risk of pancreatic cancer. Maintaining a healthy weight can be facilitated by following a nutritious diet and getting regular exercise.

A well-rounded diet

Eat a diet high in fruits, vegetables, whole grains, lean proteins, and balance to ensure optimal health. Eat less red and processed meats, as well as foods heavy in sugar and saturated fats.

Limit Your Alcohol Consumption:

There is a link between heavy and prolonged alcohol use and a higher risk of pancreatic cancer. If you decide to consume alcohol, do so sparingly.

Frequent Exercise:

Take part in regular exercise. Maintaining a healthy weight, increasing general fitness, and lowering the risk of specific cancers are just a few of the many health advantages of exercise.

Reduce Your Exposure to Workplace Risks:

There have been suggestions that certain occupational exposures, such as those to specific chemicals and pesticides, may pose a risk for pancreatic cancer. Reduce your exposure to these risks as much as you can.

Manage Diabetes:

People with diabetes, particularly those with type 2 diabetes, may be more likely to develop pancreatic cancer. Reducing this risk may be possible by managing diabetes with medication, dietary changes, and routine checkups.

Handle Persistent Pancreatitis:

Pancreatic inflammation associated with chronic pancreatitis may raise the risk of pancreatic cancer. It can be crucial to treat the underlying causes and seek medical assistance for any symptoms.

Genetic Testing and Counseling:

Genetic testing and counseling may be beneficial for people with a family history of pancreatic cancer or specific genetic syndromes. Surveillance and preventive measures can be guided by knowledge of genetic risks.

Frequent Health Check-Ups:

As advised by medical professionals, get regular checkups and screenings. For some conditions, early identification and treatment can improve results.

Minimize Your Carcinogen Exposure:

When at all possible, reduce your exposure to environmental carcinogens. This involves limiting needless exposure to chemicals and other contaminants that raise the risk of cancer.

Remain Up to Date:

Learn about the symptoms, risk factors, and preventative measures associated with pancreatic cancer. General health can be improved by being proactive and aware of the possible risks.

It is crucial to stress that different risk factors have different effects and that no single lifestyle modification can ensure the prevention of pancreatic cancer. Furthermore, it's possible that some risk factors—like genetics and family history—cannot be changed. On the other hand, combining a number of healthy living habits can improve general health and lower the risk of several cancers, including pancreatic cancer. Frequent consultations with medical professionals can offer tailored advice depending on each patient's unique health status and risk factors.

Effects on Emotion and Psychology

Pancreatic cancer diagnosis can have a significant emotional and psychological impact on the patient as well as their loved ones. Treatment for pancreatic cancer can be difficult, and the disease is frequently discovered at an advanced stage. Comprehensive care for pancreatic cancer patients requires an understanding of and attention to the psychological and emotional aspects of the disease. Here are some crucial things to remember:

Astonishment and Deflation:

A diagnosis of pancreatic cancer can be debilitating and overwhelming. When individuals and their families learn of the diagnosis, they could first feel shocked or in denial.

Anxiety and Fear:

Anxiety can be increased by a number of factors, including worries about the course of treatment, the severity of the illness, and fear of the unknown. Future uncertainty could be especially difficult.

Depression

Suffering from a severe illness such as pancreatic cancer can result in depressive symptoms. The effects on relationships, day-to-day activities, and future plans could make one feel hopeless.

Sadness and Loss:

Grief and a sense of loss for the life they had imagined before receiving a cancer diagnosis may be experienced by individuals and their families. Adapting to the psychological and physiological effects of treatment can exacerbate depressive symptoms.

CHAPTER FIVE

Relationship Stress:

Relationships with family, friends, and caregivers may be strained as a result of the psychological effects of pancreatic cancer. Relationship strain can result from difficulties in communication and managing caregiving responsibilities.

Handling Side Effects of Treatment:

Emotional well-being can be impacted by the psychological and physiological side effects of cancer treatments like chemotherapy and surgery. Emotionally taxing experiences include adjusting to pain, exhaustion, nausea, and physical changes.

Effect on Self-Image:

Surgical procedures, like the Whipple procedure, can alter the way the body looks. Managing changes in body image can have an impact on one's emotional health and sense of self.

How to Handle an Uncertain Prognosis:

Anxiety about the future and a feeling of vulnerability can be exacerbated by the frequently unclear prognosis of pancreatic cancer. It can be emotionally taxing to deal with life expectancy uncertainty.

Existential and Spiritual Issues:

When faced with a serious illness, people may struggle with existential and spiritual issues as they look for meaning and purpose in life. A key component of holistic care is addressing existential and spiritual issues.

Counseling and Support Services:

Joining a support group or going to counseling can offer emotional support and a secure environment in which to vent emotions. Professional counselors and support group members can offer insights and coping strategies.

Palliative Care and Hospice Support:

Palliative care focuses on improving the quality of life for individuals with serious illnesses, addressing physical and emotional needs.

Hospice support, when appropriate, provides compassionate care at the end of life.

Encouraging Open Communication:

Encouraging open communication within the healthcare team, as well as with family and friends, allows individuals to voice their emotional issues and get support.

Providing Education:

Providing information and education about pancreatic cancer, treatment options, and expected problems can enable individuals to navigate their emotional journey with a better awareness of what to expect.

Creating a Supportive Environment:

Creating a supportive environment that recognizes and supports emotional experiences is vital. This includes including loved ones in the caring process and establishing open communication.

Addressing the emotional and psychological consequences of pancreatic cancer demands a broad and supportive approach. Healthcare practitioners, mental health specialists, and supportive care teams play crucial roles in assisting individuals and their loved ones negotiate the emotional problems associated with the disease. Additionally, creating a supporting network and finding community services might contribute to a more resilient mental well-being during the cancer journey.

Pancreatic cancer is a difficult adversary, offering considerable obstacles due to its generally late-stage diagnosis and aggressive nature. The complexity of this disease underlines the necessity of continued research, early identification efforts, and breakthroughs in treatment approaches. While progress has been made in understanding pancreatic cancer, much remains to be done to improve outcomes and better the quality of life for those affected.

The path through pancreatic cancer needs a multidisciplinary approach, including surgical treatments, chemotherapy, radiation therapy, and supportive care. Each individual's experience is unique, and tailored treatment strategies are required to suit the specific conditions of the disease.

Emotionally, pancreatic cancer takes a toll on individuals and their loved ones. Coping with the shock of diagnosis, negotiating treatment decisions, and facing the uncertainty of prognosis can be stressful. Emotional and psychological care, including counseling and support groups, plays a significant role in meeting the holistic needs of persons impacted by pancreatic cancer.

Survivorship, when achieved, brings with it continuous problems and the need for vigilant monitoring for potential recurrence or late consequences of treatment. Creating a supportive atmosphere, both inside the hospital system and in the larger community, is vital for persons transitioning into the post-treatment period.

Preventive methods, such as lifestyle adjustments and early detection campaigns, contribute to the collective efforts aimed at reducing the incidence of pancreatic cancer. These strategies, together with current research into risk factors and genetic predispositions, hold promise for improving outcomes and lowering the burden of this disease.

In conclusion, the war against pancreatic cancer demands a comprehensive and interdisciplinary approach. From early detection and treatment improvements to emotional support and survivorship care, every part of the journey plays a key role in the drive for better outcomes and, ultimately, a future where pancreatic cancer is more successfully controlled and, one day, conquered.

THE END